The Bett Back Guide

By S.J. White

LONDON : HMSO

ISBN 0 11 701846 5

My sincere thanks to:

Brenda Noonan

Nicola Murphy

Patrick Tomlin

Jonathan Regan

-INDEX-

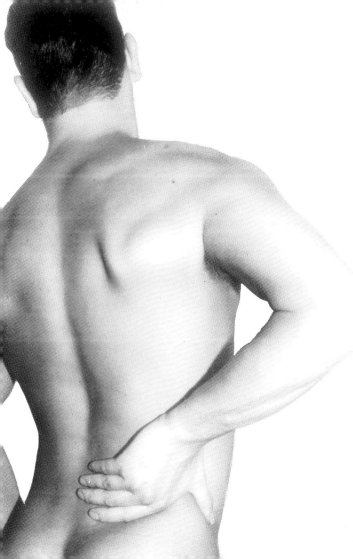

THE BETTER BACK GUIDE

Back pain can strike at anyone of any age and at any time. There are over 90,000 people a day in this country alone who are unable to attend their place of work due to back pain!

Statistics show there is an increase in the number of people suffering from some form or other back related problems. Over 30 million working days are lost each year as a result of bad backs. With such a vast number of the population suffering from back pain, we here at "Your Fitness" decided on a closer look at this vast problem. "The Better Back Guide" will, we believe, give you a greater understanding of the mechanics of the back. In addition the step by step guide on how you can bring about improvement and relief through remedial exercises is designed to help your spine regain both strength and flexibility.

BACK PAIN

It is important that if you have, or have had, experience of back pain you must always consult your doctor and/or your osteopath *(always make sure the latter is registered)*. By giving them a precise idea of exactly where you feel the pain and what brought about the problem they will be able to diagnose the correct treatment.

Back pain is brought about by such a variety of reasons: lifting incorrectly/accidents/bad habits in one's posture/sports injuries/sedentary life style and sometimes through bad maintenance! Yes bad maintenance! If some people took as much care of their back as they do their motor car the shocking statistics on back trouble in this country would be halved! But let us take the scenario one step further. How many of us would expect a lifetime of use out of one motor car? Not too many of us, especially without proper maintenance.

With the many reasons and causes that lead to back pain it is important that we understand that there are ways to bring about positive results and improvement. With this book we outline a number of ways to bring relief, plus a complete range of exercises to help maintain flexibility in your back to ensure a lifetime's use.

Now let us take a closer look at the back's structure.

To do this I will divide the spine itself into two groups, the first is the Lower Back *(Lumbar Spine)*, and the second naturally is the Upper Back *(Thoracic Spine)*. To start I want us to take a detailed look at our Lower Back.

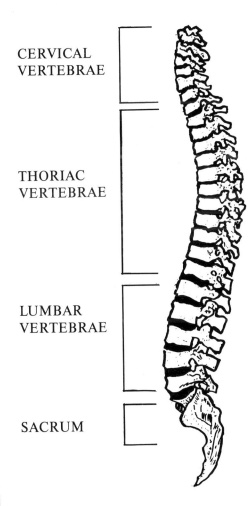

CERVICAL
VERTEBRAE

THORIAC
VERTEBRAE

LUMBAR
VERTEBRAE

SACRUM

THE LUMBAR SPINE :

Its structure

The lumbar spine is the lowest part of your back and curves forward to form a hollow above your pelvis. It consists of five bony vertebrae, which are all linked together by ligaments and muscles and soft tissue discs between the bones.

Each one of the five bones is in a form of a cylindrical block which is backed by a triangular structure of finer bones. Each triangle of bone has a short strut of bone protruding upwards, downwards and to each side. The vertical struts interlink with the upward and downward struts on the vertebrae, above and below, to form very closely knitted joints.

The backward and sideways struts also form joints with the equivalent fine bones on the vertebrae above and below. These also are linked by ligaments, but the bones in each joint are not so close together. You can actually feel the struts which project backwards from the vertebrae. These form the spine which run the whole length of your back. You can see them through the skin.

LUMBAR VERTEBRAE

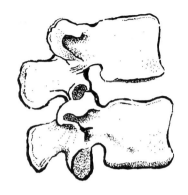

ANTERIOR LONGITUDINAL LIGAMENT

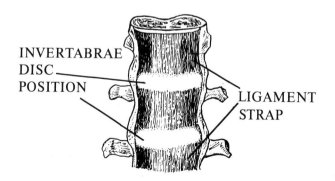

INVERTABRAE DISC POSITION

LIGAMENT STRAP

However it would be harder to feel the sideways struts, as these are covered by the spine's thick mass of muscle and again, the vertical struts are sited equally deeply in the lower trunk and harder to feel.

The lowest of the lumbar vertebrae, known technically as L5, lies on top of the sacrum. It is flat and cylindrical in shape to correspond to the block bone forming the main body of the L5 vertebra. The body of L5 is just slightly longer at the front than at the back of the block to help form the forward curve of the lumbar pelvis. Please note there are different degrees of curvature in the lumbar spine, so the actual shape of L5 and the rest of the other wedge shaped vertebrae will vary from person to person.

So if we think of the spine as being a series of blocks placed vertically one on top of the other we won't be far wrong. The ligament joining these series of blocks is also more or less vertical. This is a very strong ligament which runs the length of the spine and is attached to the front of each vertical block. It is called the **ANTERIOR LONGITUDINAL LIGAMENT**. This ligament forms a long strap, binding all the vertebrae together, from the top of the skull right down to the top of the front of the sacrum.

A similar ligament runs the length of the vertebrae across the back of the vertebra blocks, from the top of the sacrum, up as far as the second vertebra in the neck. Please note there are no ligaments at the sides of the vertebrae bodies. Short strong ligaments bind together the struts of bone on the fine arches at the back of the vertebrae. Here the vertical struts lie close together to form their joints. The ligament binding the sideways and backwards struts are attached vertically between the corresponding bones on each vertebra. One long ligament covers the tips of the backward spine spreading vertically from the lowest of the neck vertebrae to the top of the sacrum.

THE DISCS

The discs in the spine are the connecting structures which lie between the bodies of the vertebrae. The discs fit neatly into the flat surfaces forming both top and bottom of each vertebral section. You have a disc between each vertebra, running up from the top of the sacrum and L5 *(lowest lumbar vertebra),* right up to the joint between the third and second vertebra in the neck. They actually make up approximately one fifth of the length of the spine. However the thickness and size of the individual discs does vary; they are much thicker in the lumbar region compared to the thoracic region (upper back) directly above the lumbar.

The structure of the discs: Each disc is welded or stuck between each vertebra, and its construction has two main features. The easiest way to describe these is to liken them to a raw egg. In the very centre of the disc *(like the yellow yoke of an egg)* is the *"Nucleus pulposes"* which is a waterfilled transparent jelly. This nucleus is very pliable, almost elastic in the very young, but it does gradually become harder as one ages. This is due to the loss of its water holding capacity. The centre of the disc is 90% water at birth but by the time a person reaches the age of sixty-five years it's only approximately 70% water.

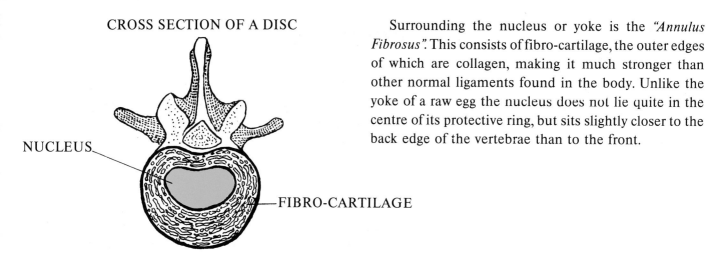

CROSS SECTION OF A DISC

NUCLEUS

FIBRO-CARTILAGE

Surrounding the nucleus or yoke is the *"Annulus Fibrosus"*. This consists of fibro-cartilage, the outer edges of which are collagen, making it much stronger than other normal ligaments found in the body. Unlike the yoke of a raw egg the nucleus does not lie quite in the centre of its protective ring, but sits slightly closer to the back edge of the vertebrae than to the front.

THE LOWER BACK'S FUNCTION

Only slight movements take place between individual vertebrae, due to the way the bone structure interlocks. However, the combined movements of the whole spine do allow quite a good range of movement. Your abdominal muscles pull your spine forwards while the long extension muscles pull your spine backwards; you are able to bend from side to side through the contraction of the oblique muscles on the side of your trunk and you can twist from side to side due to the action of the small rotor muscles in your back that work in synchronization with the diagonal abdominal muscles. The movements in the lumbar spine, both bending backwards and sideways, are the lower back's least restricted movements. Forward bending is much more limited and the twisting of the lower spine is restricted.

THE MECHANICS

You should think of your spine acting as a series of mobile levers when you bend or twist or as a rigid single lever when you brace your back i.e. when you prepare to lift up a weight. In all forms of sport as well as throughout our everyday life our spine provides mobility and power. Consider, if you will, some of the force both our spines and discs take. Remember the spine has to cope with, and absorb, shock and compressing forces including the earth's gravity.

When you jump down from a height or fall and land on your head, the force of the impact has to be absorbed by the discs. If this force is too great you can smash one or more of your discs, even crush some of the vertebrae. It must be said that normal discs have a great resilience, but remember that this does become undermined as one becomes older or if you have previously injured your back. The vertebrae also play a protective role. The spinal cord is enclosed within the bony arches found at the back of the spine. This cord extends right down from the brain to the second lumbar vertebra and is an important part of your central nervous system and never heals if damaged.

At the point of each vertabrae, tiny little nerves lead off from the spinal cord. These in turn form part of your peripheral nervous system which gives the sensation and motor power right around your body. The nerves from the lumbar spine also supply your legs.

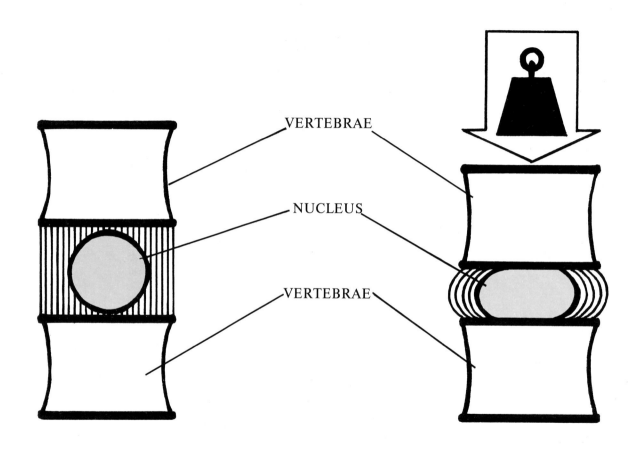

VERTEBRAE

NUCLEUS

VERTEBRAE

NORMAL POSITION OF DISC

DISC UNDER SHOCK PRESSURE

YOUR POSTURE

This is so important we will discuss it here as well as in the exercise programme, covered later, which is designed to further improve your posture. Your posture in your lumbar spine is influenced by a variety of factors: your personal patterns of movement; the positions you adopt; the way you lift/hold/carry weight etc; not forgetting the force of gravity! If we adopt a **GOOD** posture that holds our trunks and limbs in correct alignment, we will minimise strain on both joints and soft tissues. Bad posture is one of the root causes of back pain! We must remember that our lumbar spine is supposed to curve forwards. Slouching or twisting lead to strain. You have to train yourself to get into good habits. Trying to keep a symmetrical posture whilst not forgetting your pelvis and shoulders affect and influence your lower back.

THE UPPER BACK :
The Thoracic Spine

The upper part of the back is called the thorax. This extends from slightly above the waistline to the level of the shoulders and consists of twelve thoracic vertebrae and the rib cage. The ribs are attached on either side of your vertebrae at your back and again at your breast bone in your chest. This forms a rounded bony container giving protection to the vital organs. The thoracic vertebra are similar in both construction and form to the lumbar vertebra, in that they have a main block of bone with fine struts forming a fine arch projecting from the back of it.

THORACIC VERTEBRAE

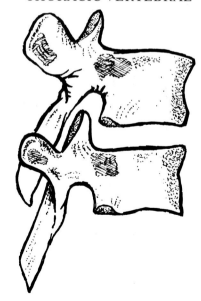

The thoracic bones differ from the lumbar in detail. They are smaller and tend to be wedge-shaped; they also taper forward so that the front edge of the block is more shallow than the back. The joints at the sides of the arches are not interlocked in the same way as the lumbar spine's vertebrae, the thoracic bones are joined together by ligaments again joining each ligament in line. The bodies of the vertebrae are held by the same long bands which extend up to the front and back of the bones. The struts of the arches are all bound to the struts on the vertebrae both above and below with finer ligaments whilst the bones which are close enough on adjacent arches form joints bound in their retaining, fluid filled, capsules. Each vertebral body is separated and cushioned from the next by a disc, which as we mentioned earlier, is much thinner than the discs found in your lumbar region *(Lower Back)*.

The main difference between the thoracic and lumbar vertebrae is that the thoracic bones form a joint with the ribs. The ends of the ribs fit into a notch on either side of the vertebral bodies and are held there by a retaining capsule.

Apart from your eleventh and twelfth ribs *(which are short)* all your other ribs form a joint with the sideways struts from the vertebral arches. If we look at where the ribs connect to the spine we will see they are as if held in two clamps to the thoracic vertebrae. The ribs extend away from these attachments to enclose your chest cavity. The thoracic spine forms a central pillar from which your ribs arch away symmetrically on either side forming the vital protection for your organs.

With most people, the spines of the thoracic vertebrae stand out prominently, as it is this part of the vertebral column which curves backwards. When you bend over with a mirror behind you, you can see the spines outlined through the skin.

THE UPPER BACK'S FUNCTION

Due to the spines at the back of the thoracic overlapping closely in a backward direction there is very little leeway for any backward movement in this part of your spine. Forward movement is also very limited, due to both your ligaments and the shape of your thoracic bones. The ability to twist is the least restricted movement in this part of your spine. The movements are achieved through the co-ordination between the complex muscles lining your spine and the muscles positioned around your trunk.

We must remember that all the movement in the spinal column is interlinked so it is not possible to separate movement in one region from another, nor can you achieve any active movement at all in an isolated reaction between two vertebrae. The functional co-ordination between all your vertebrae means that the spine allows a good range of movements, as well as its shock-absorbing and protective functions. In the thoracic region, the bones form a part of the protective ring around your lungs and heart. The twisting movement allowed by your thoracic spine is essential to all daily activities from sports to housework.

The thoracic spine like the rest of the body is subject to the compressive pressure of gravity.

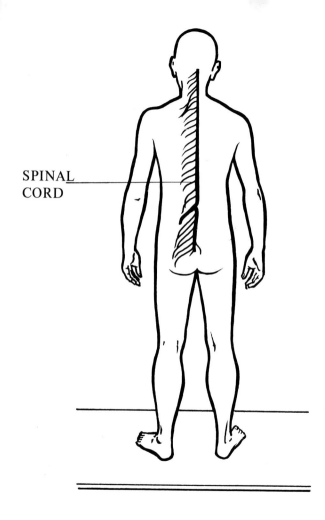

SPINAL
CORD

THE SPINAL CORD

At birth the spinal cord extends from the base of your brain to your sacrum. Due to the uneven growth rate of the spine, it runs only to your first lumbar vertebra by the time you are in your early teens. All the nerves branch out from the spine at this point. All the nerve roots leave the immediate area of the spinal cord and move out to merge with other nerve roots. Some of these nerves merge to assist in providing muscular co-ordination and motor skills, whilst others carry pain sensations or go to the skin or other organs.

For example, the fourth and fifth lumbar vertebra nerve roots and the first three sacral nerve roots combine to form the two sciatic nerves, the thickest nerves in the body. One sciatic nerve goes all the way down the back of each leg. It divides at the back of your knee, where one branch travels down your shin into the big toe, and the other runs down the back of your calf to the heel before winding around to the front of your foot and into your toes.

The entire nervous system has so many branches it is impossible to measure them all accurately.

THE COLUMN OF LIFE

From the previous pages we now know what the spine consists of and how it functions. But what does a healthy back mean to you and me? Quite simply, the ability to live a normal active life. Like the wise words of a song *"You'll never know what you have got until it's gone"* this is unfortunately the case with most people who develop back problems.

We all take our health pretty much for granted in our youth when our spines are supple and flexible. As we grow older, however, we stiffen up, generally as a result of a combination of misuse/bad posture and failure to keep flexible.

This book is designed to bring relief from back pain in the case of back pain sufferers and bring remedial help to those with sports injuries.

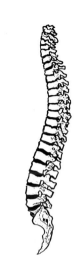

BEFORE YOU START . . . !

IT IS MOST IMPORTANT THAT, IF YOU SUFFER FROM EITHER CHRONIC OR RECURRING BACK PAIN, YOU SHOULD REVIEW THIS EXERCISE PROGRAMME WITH YOUR DOCTOR.

Your doctor may wish to change the format to suit your own personal condition. Remembering that each and every person will vary from one another, this book is a guide and does not represent the only approach to back pain prevention and relief. If any new pain or other symptoms show themselves either during or after this exercise programme, do not use it further without consulting your doctor. Read and absorb all the material before you begin the exercise programme.

THE EXERCISE PROGRAMME

The exercises are split into group types:

GROUP ONE:

These exercises are designed for people who are not used to exercising and are just starting to get their spines flexible once again. All the exercise illustrations for group one are coloured pink. We shall aim to stretch areas of the spine not normally exercised in daily activities. It is important, therefore, that Group One ONLY DO THE EXERCISES WHICH ARE COLOURED PINK.

GROUP TWO: ⃠

These are more or less the same exercises as the previous group but slightly more advanced, most of you will become much more flexible as you progress. **But remember don't run before you can walk! The name of the game is improvement and to aim to develop further flexibility in your spine.** Group Two can do ALL THE EXERCISES ILLUSTRATED.

I want you to make this exercise programme part of your everyday routine, use it and perform the exercises correctly. Make sure you do the exercises slowly and smoothly. Don't rush and avoid all jerky quick movements and don't over stretch. You will no doubt experience some tightness during some of the exercises but this is nothing to worry about. However, if any exercise causes either a sharp pain or tingling in your back or legs, stop the exercise!

POINTS TO REMEMBER

1. **MAKE THE EXERCISES PART OF YOUR DAILY ROUTINE.**

2. **ALWAYS TRY AND WARM UP BEFORE YOU START YOUR EXERCISES.**
   (Either by walking around the house or by taking a hot bath or shower).

3. **FIND A COMFORTABLE PLACE TO EXERCISE.**
   You will need a mat, blanket or thick towel. Avoid very hard surfaces if possible. And keep yourself warm.

4. **DO ALL THE EXERCISES SLOWLY AND CORRECTLY, DON'T RUSH!**

5. **FINISH THE EXERCISE ROUTINE WITH 5 MINUTES RELAXATION.**

6. **DO NOT HOLD YOUR BREATH WHILE EXERCISING. MAKE IT A HABIT TO BREATHE DEEPLY AS YOU START EACH EXERCISE, THEN MAINTAIN A CONTROLLED RHYTHM OF BREATHING THROUGHOUT EACH OF THE EXERCISES.**

7. **DON'T EXERCISE IF YOU FEEL UNWELL, OR TIRED.**

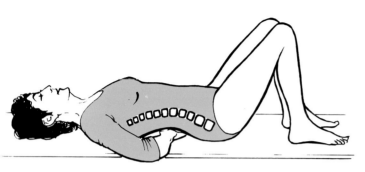

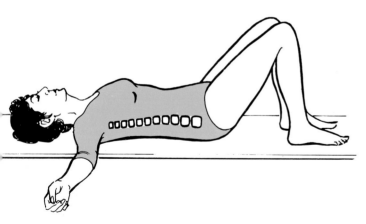

THE PELVIC TILT

(Both groups complete this exercise please)

EXECUTION: Lie on your back with your knees bent and your head comfortably supported. Place your hand down to the small of your back and feel the slight arch in your lower back. We are going to press this arch down to meet the floor. This helps to reduce the stress on your lower back. Squeeze your buttocks together, tighten your abdominal muscles, then raise your backside slightly off the floor until the small of your back is pressing flat against the floor. **HOLD THIS POSITION FOR THE COUNT OF TEN SECONDS.**

Relax, place your hand once again to the small of your back and feel the arch in your spine.

REPEAT THIS EXERCISE THREE TIMES.

THERAPEUTIC EFFECT: This exercise tilts the pelvic region and reduces the stress on your lower back. By rotating the pelvic bone it decreases the curve in the lower part of your spine. This exercise will aid good posture.

THE SINGLE KNEE TO CHEST

(Group One)

EXECUTION: Still in the lying position, bring the right knee up **(See illustration)** clasp both hands together around your right knee and pull towards your chest. Make sure both your head and your shoulders remain on the floor. **HOLD THIS POSITION FOR THE COUNT OF TEN SECONDS.**

Returning slowly to the start position, rest. Then repeat the exercise with the left knee. Again, hold for the count of ten seconds. Repeat this exercise once more on each leg.

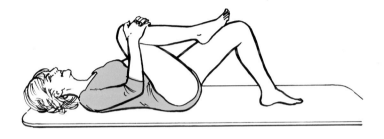

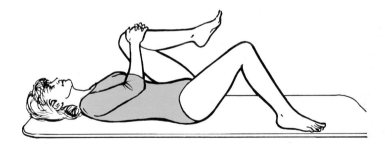

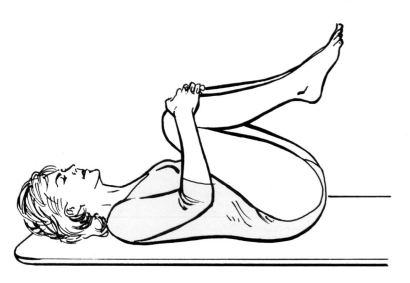

BOTH KNEES TO CHEST

(Group Two)

This exercise as you can see is basically the same as its predecessor. The important thing to remember is not to bring both knees up at the same time.

EXECUTION: Pull your right knee towards your chest and hold it there, then pull your left knee towards your chest. Clasp both hands together and pull your knees down towards your chest, as close as you can. You will feel the stretch in your lower back, your backside will raise slightly off the floor. **HOLD THIS POSITION FOR THE COUNT OF FIFTEEN SECONDS.**

Returning to the start position, rest. Then repeat this exercise once more, again, hold for the count of **FIFTEEN SECONDS.**

THERAPEUTIC EFFECT: This exercise stretches the muscles in both the hips and buttocks.

THE SPINAL STRETCH

(Both Groups do this exercise please)

WE RECOMMEND THAT YOU USE A FEW BOOKS TO ACT AS A WEIGHT. A COUPLE OF TELEPHONE DIRECTORIES ARE IDEAL.

EXECUTION: Lie on your back keeping your knees bent and your back flat against the floor **(See illustration).** Tighten the muscles underneath your bottom. Then slowly stretch your arms above your head to lengthen your upper back. Grasp hold of the books to weigh your hands down and then slowly stretch as far as you can. You will feel the muscles in your abdomen tighten as your stomach flattens. Still retaining the stretch, slowly straighten your legs down to the floor, remembering to keep the lower back flat to the floor throughout the exercise.

HOLD THIS POSITION FOR TWENTY SECONDS. *(Group One).*

GROUP TWO MAY HOLD THE POSITION FOR AS LONG AS YOU CAN *(feeling comfortable).*

REMEMBER TO BREATHE NORMALLY THROUGHOUT THIS EXERCISE.

THERAPEUTIC EFFECT: This exercise will help stretch the muscles which are over-used and become tight through sitting and walking. Also the lengthening and stretching will benefit the spine.

Position 1

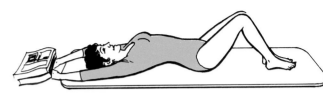

Position 2

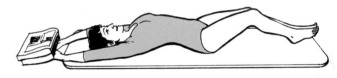

Position 3

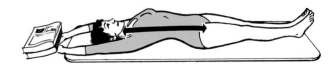

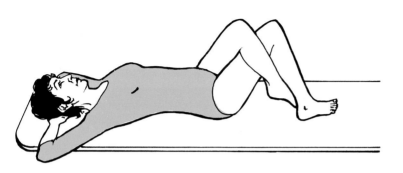

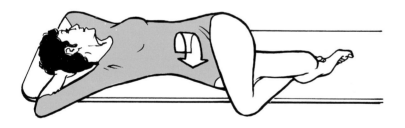

THE TRUNK TWIST

(Both Groups do this exercise please)

EXECUTION: Place your hands behind your head in a comfortable position with your elbows outstretched, then slowly bring your knees up **(See illustration).** Now slowly cross your left knee over your right thigh. Take a deep breath and slowly let the weight of your left leg push down your left knee towards the floor. As your leg moves down slowly turn your head towards your left shoulder. Making sure your shoulders remain flat on the floor with your hands still clasped behind your head, stretch as far as is comfortable and hold. **HOLD THE POSITION FOR BETWEEN TEN AND FIFTEEN SECONDS.** Then slowly return to the start position and relax.

Now repeat the exercise on the opposite side. This time crossing your right knee over your left thigh and allowing the weight of your right leg to slowly push down towards your left side. Remember to slowly turn your head to the right. Please also remember to let your knees drop as close to the floor as you can. **BUT NEVER STRETCH TO THE POINT OF PAIN!**

AGAIN, HOLD THIS POSITION FOR TEN TO FIFTEEN SECONDS.

REPEAT THIS EXERCISE ONCE MORE EACH SIDE.

THERAPEUTIC EFFECT: This exercise both stretches and strengthens the muscles in the lower back and each side of the abdomen and helps maintain spinal flexibility.

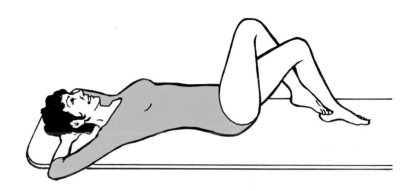

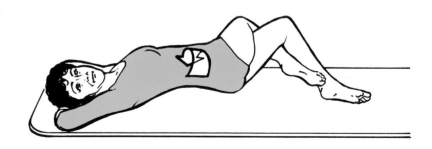

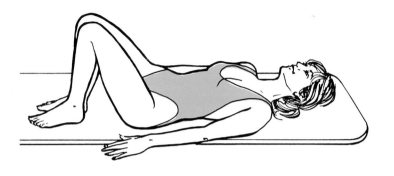

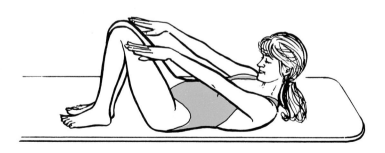

THE ABDOMINAL CRAMP

(Variations in both Group One and Group Two)

GROUP ONE:

EXECUTION: Lying on the floor with both arms straight out in front of you **(See illustration)** slowly bring your knees up and together into a sit-up position. Lift your bottom slightly off the floor and flatten the arch of your back to the floor; *(Pelvic Tilt),* tuck your chin onto your chest and slowly lift both your head and shoulders off the floor using your arms as a counter balance and pointing your hands to the top of your knees. **HOLD THIS POSITION FOR THE COUNT OF FIVE SECONDS.** Slowly lower yourself back to the floor and relax completely before you continue.

GROUP TWO: May place their hands behind their heads and hold exercise for **SEVEN SECONDS.**

BOTH GROUPS REPEAT EXERCISE TWICE MORE.

REMEMBER DO NOT HOLD YOUR BREATH WHILE DOING THIS EXERCISE, BREATHE NORMALLY.

THERAPEUTIC EFFECT: The Abdominal Cramp and the Cross-Over Abdominal Cramp both help strengthen the abdominal muscles. Weak abdominal muscles not only promote bad posture but also upset the balance between the way the abdominals and spinal erectors hold the spine upright, much the same way as guy lines hold and support a tent pole.

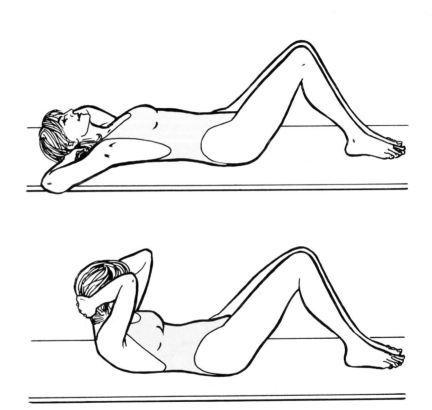

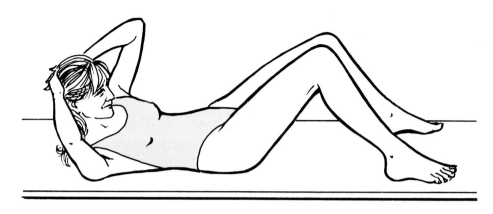

THE CROSS-OVER ABDOMINAL CRAMP

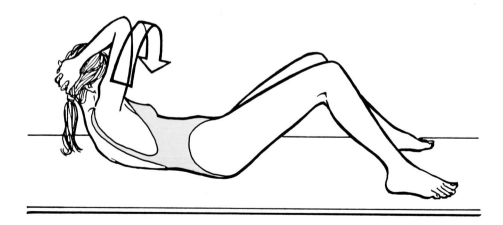

THE CROSS-OVER ABDOMINAL CRAMP

(Group Two only please)

EXECUTION: This exercise is very similar to the last. Bring your legs up together but keep your feet about 18 inches (450 millimetres) apart. Flatten the arch of your back to the floor (*(Pelvic Tilt)* and place your hands behind your head. Now slowly lift your right shoulder off the floor and rotate your elbow and shoulder towards the left **(See illustration). HOLD THIS POSITION FOR FIVE SECONDS.** Then slowly return to the starting position. Relax completely before repeating the exercise. Only this time reverse the procedure with the left shoulder coming up off the floor and rotating to the right. **AGAIN HOLD THIS POSITION FOR FIVE SECONDS.** Slowly lower yourself down and relax completely before you continue.

REPEAT EXERCISE TWICE MORE.

**PLEASE BE AWARE OF YOUR BREATHING DURING THIS EXERCISE
AND DON'T HOLD YOUR BREATH!**

THE COBRA POSTURE

(Both Groups complete this exercise please)

This is a yoga exercise and took its name from the snake. If you look at the diagram you can see the similarity in the position when the cobra raises its head.

EXECUTION: Lying with your stomach pressed flat on the floor, place both of your hands, palms down, in front of you, just below your shoulders. Take a deep breath and slowly raise your head back as far as you can, placing your awareness to your lower back and tightening your muscles in this region. Now, using your arms to push away slowly lift your shoulders making sure your tummy remains pressed firmly to the floor. **HOLD THIS POSITION FOR FIVE SECONDS** *(Group One)* : **SEVEN SECONDS** *(Group Two)*. Slowly come out of the exercise and relax fully before repeating this exercise twice more.

THERAPEUTIC EFFECT: This exercise helps to overcome stiffness in the lower back, and as blood is forced to all the nerves in the region it is beneficial to the whole nervous system. The Cobra helps strengthen the lower back and improve both mobility and posture.

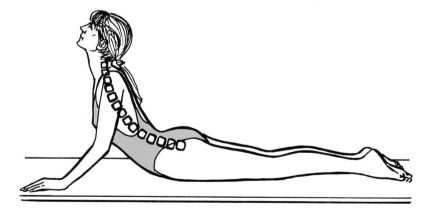

THE CAT

(Both Groups complete this exercise please)

This is another exercise based on yoga, again taken from the cat. Watch a cat raise itself from slumber and stretch its back fully.

EXECUTION: Assume the position **(See illustration).** Hands placed at shoulder width and keeping your knees about eight inches (200 millimetres) apart. Then slowly arch your back up and lower your head tucking your chin into your chest. Tighten your abdominal muscles as you hold the posture. **HOLD THIS POSITION FOR THE COUNT OF FIVE SECONDS** *(Group One)*: **GROUP TWO HOLD THIS POSITION FOR THE COUNT OF TEN SECONDS.**

Slowly come out of the stretch, letting your head lift up. Imagine you are pushing your stomach towards the floor and pointing your head up to the ceiling **(See illustration).** Once your head is raised and you are facing ahead, push your bottom up and out. **HOLD THIS POSITION FOR THE COUNT OF FIVE SECONDS** *(Group One)* : **GROUP TWO HOLD POSITION FOR TEN SECONDS. REPEAT THIS EXERCISE TWICE MORE.**

THERAPEUTIC EFFECT: The Cat chases away stiffness and brings flexibility to the whole spine.

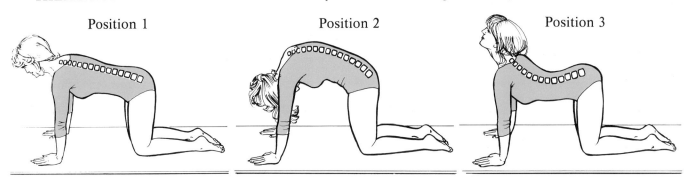

Position 1   Position 2   Position 3

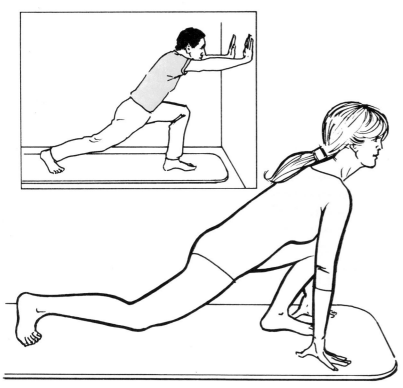

THE HALF LUNGE
(Variations in both Group One and Group Two)

This exercise like the previous two, is also based on yoga. The exercise in essence stretches the hip/groin and muscles of the inner thigh.

GROUP ONE: First find a wall with enough space for you to stretch out, making quite sure both the wall and the floor nearby are not slippery or damaged and offer good support and traction.

EXECUTION: Place your hands shoulder width apart, palms facing the wall. Lean into the wall and place your right leg back keeping your weight on the ball of your left foot **(See illustration).** Now slowly bring your left leg forward and push gently against the wall, feeling the stretch. **HOLD THIS POSITION FOR TEN SECONDS.** Come back to the start position and repeat the exercise but this time bring your left leg back etc. **AGAIN, HOLD THIS POSITION FOR TEN SECONDS.**

REPEAT THIS EXERCISE TWICE MORE.

GROUP TWO: Kneel with your left knee on the floor and your right foot forward, keeping your shin in a vertical position. Take a deep breath, breathe out and shift your weight from your left knee to the right foot. Now push your left leg back whilst slowly lowering the trunk until your hands touch the floor. The back must be held upright **(See illustration)** you will feel this stretch mainly in the groin region. **HOLD THIS POSITION FOR BETWEEN FOUR AND SEVEN SECONDS.** Then rise slowly and take a deep breath before returning to the start position.

REPEAT THIS TWICE MORE THEN CHANGE FEET.

THERAPEUTIC EFFECT: This exercise improves flexibility of the legs, hips, hamstrings and helps banish fatty deposits in the hip region.

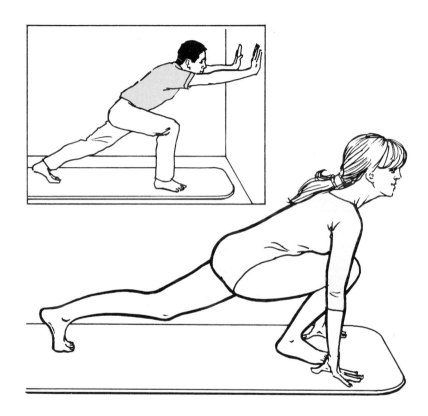

THE CHILD POSTURE

(Both Groups complete this exercise please)

You may use a pillow or cushion if you are unable to touch your head to the floor. This is one of my favourite exercises. The Child Posture is a symbol of yoga.

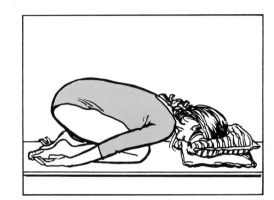

EXECUTION: Kneel on the floor with your bottom resting on your heels. Your knees should be approximately twelve inches (305mm) apart forming a "V" shape.

Take a deep breath. Then slowly bend forward whilst breathing out, letting your head touch the floor, putting your hands down by your side. **HOLD THIS POSITION FOR BETWEEN TEN AND THIRTY SECONDS, THEN SLOWLY BREATHE IN AND COME SLOWLY OUT OF THE EXERCISE AND STRAIGHTEN UP AND RELAX.**

THERAPEUTIC EFFECT:
This exercise both stretches the back and helps to develop strong abdominal muscles.

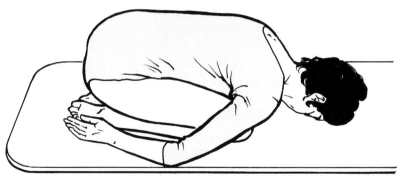

THE HURDLER'S STRETCH

(Both Groups complete this exercise please)

This exercise takes its name from the athletes who put it to most use. It is a great exercise for stretching the muscles in the back of your thighs "The Hamstrings".

EXECUTION: Sitting on the floor straighten your right leg in front of you. Keeping the leg as straight as possible with your knee firmly on the ground and your foot straight, toes pointing up, place your left foot into your right knee **(See illustration)**. Now very slowly, bend forward, reaching out with both hands as far as you can without any pain. **HOLD THIS POSITION FOR BETWEEN FIVE AND TEN SECONDS.** Then slowly return to the starting position and relax. Reverse the exercise by switching legs. **AGAIN, HOLD THIS POSITION FOR BETWEEN FIVE AND TEN SECONDS. REPEAT ONCE MORE EACH LEG.**

THERAPEUTIC EFFECT: This exercise stretches the hamstrings and brings flexibility to the knees.

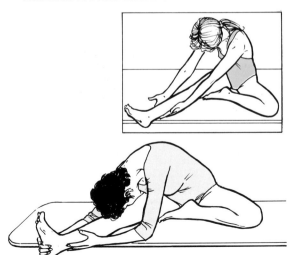

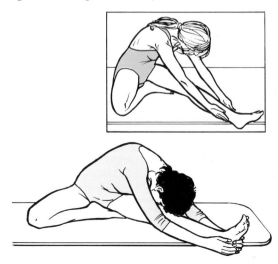

THE SQUAT

(Both Groups complete this exercise please)

This is another great exercise with many benefits for the whole body.

WE RECOMMEND THAT A BOOK BE PLACED BENEATH THE HEELS AND A CHAIR BE USED AS AN AID TO BALANCE FOR THOSE NEW TO THIS EXERCISE.

EXECUTION: In a standing position, feet approximately shoulder width apart, tighten both the abdominal muscles and those in your bottom. Keeping your back straight and your head facing forward, slowly lower yourself into the squat position. Go down as far as you can without causing any pain. **HOLD THIS POSITION FOR BETWEEN FIVE AND TEN SECONDS (BOTH GROUPS).** Now slowly stand up straight. Rest before you go on to complete the exercise twice more.

THERAPEUTIC EFFECT: The Squat is an exercise which will strengthen the muscles in your thighs and bottom. It will help also improve both your posture and balance.

ONCE YOU HAVE COMPLETED ALL THE EXERCISES FIND A COMFORTABLE SPOT AND LIE ON THE FLOOR ON YOUR BACK AND RELAX FOR AT LEAST FIVE MINUTES.

THE SQUAT

START

GROUP ONE

FINISH

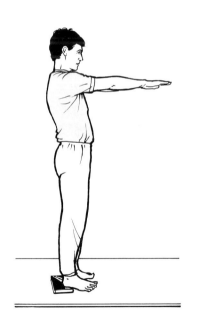

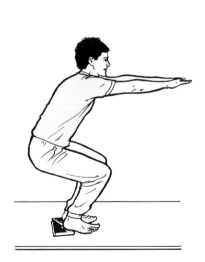

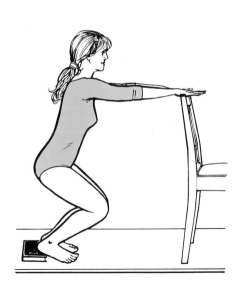

RELAXATION

So few of us these days in the hustle and rush of modern life know how to truly relax! This is a great shame putting another chink in our armour as we strive for good health.

To aid us in our relaxation we shall require a quiet room, a comfortable position on the floor and maybe a blanket to keep you warm *(you may not be able to properly relax if you become cold).*

If you have a favourite piece of music, put it on as this will also help.

POSITION: Lying on the floor let your body become aware of its contact with the flat surface, let your body press to the floor. Feel your body releasing its tension as your muscles slowly relax, letting your weight seemingly press down to the floor. Take five

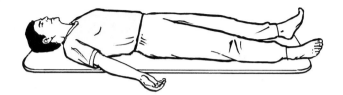

deep breaths breathing out slowly after each inhalation. Becoming aware of each breath you take and the sensation of well-being coming over you. After the fifth breath let your breathing become more relaxed and regulated. Let your mind reflect your thoughts away and concentrate just on your breathing and with every breath you take feel yourself becoming more relaxed. Close your eyes, relax and let your body rest and rejuvenate itself.

THERAPEUTIC EFFECT: Once you are able to truly take a brief segment of the day and dedicate it to relaxation, you will find improvement in the whole of your mental outlook and physical health. It is the key that unlocks so many stressful situations that we all face throughout the course of the day and will help bring both our minds and bodies back to a natural balance.

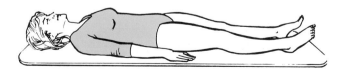

THE RULES

SURVIVAL "MIND YOUR BACKS PLEASE!"

So many back problems are brought about as a result of improper bending and reaching. We can reduce the odds substantially by simply keeping the objects we need to use most often at a level that can be reached without too much bending and stretching, i.e. between the level of your shoulders and your waist. It's a good idea to get all your wardrobe space and shelves at home organized in this way, not forgetting your place of work too. So remember, all heavier objects to be stored at a level between shoulder and waist height.

"GOING DOWN!"

Here are some points you must remember if you ever have to pick something up from or get down and clean a floor. Always lower your body by bending your knees and keeping your back straight. If you do have to get on all fours to do housework please remember not to let your back sag in the middle.

LIFTING

Again so many injuries and problems are caused by lifting things the WRONG way! We are able to reduce the risk of injury to our backs by following these simple rules.

FIRSTLY, BEFORE YOU LIFT ANYTHING:
1. **Make sure you keep your feet placed firmly on the ground, always be aware of the condition of the ground's surface, i.e. - not slippery etc.**
2. **Keep your feet shoulder width apart, with your toes pointing out slightly to provide a stable base.**
3. **Use your knees to slowly bend down to the required level of the object that you wish to lift. REMEMBER NEVER BEND FROM THE WAIST.**

4. **Always face the object you wish to lift.** Before you take the load, tighten your abdominal muscles. This will help give extra support to your spine. Keep the object that you wish to lift or carry as close to your body as you possibly can, remembering to keep the load centred. Most importantly never hold an object or weight on one side of the body!

5. **When lifting, let the strong muscles in your legs do the work.** Lift with your legs not your back! Lift slowly and steadily, do not attempt to jerk the load up as this will transfer all the load to your back! Keep the back straight at all times, remembering to keep your knees slightly bent even when you are standing (this will help keep the back straight).

These rules must be applied no matter what the weight you wish to pick up! Where possible always seek help if an object is large or cumbersome, don't attempt to lift it alone.

PLEASE SIT DOWN

Now I expect most people reading this will be sitting down at the time. The actual sitting position is very stressful for anyone with back problems. Sitting in the same position for long periods of time will aggravate most back problems, so if you must sit down for long periods of time, try changing the position in your chair every 20 minutes or so. Remember you can reduce the curve of your lower back and reduce the strain by keeping one knee higher than the level of your hips, i.e. crossing your legs. Again it is important to alternate legs frequently. Even better to put your feet up on a foot stool.

When rising from the sitting position always let your arms do most of the work in supporting your weight. It also helps to slide your bottom to the edge of the seat, making sure your feet are shoulder width apart, with one placed slightly in front of the other to aid good balance. Then lean forward and moving your shoulders over your feet use the muscles of both arms and legs to push yourself both forward and up in one single controlled motion.

Please remember to get yourself into the good habit of doing these exercise routines a minimum of three times a week. They will help you to achieve and maintain good flexibility and posture which is so essential to a happy active life style.

GOOD LUCK AND ENJOY YOUR FITNESS!

Printed in the United Kingdom for HMSO
Dd.300790 C100, 4/95, 38938